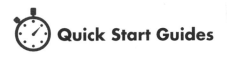 **Quick Start Guides**

The Essential

SIRT FOOD
DIET RECIPE BOOK

A Quick Start Guide To Cooking on The SIRT Food Diet!

Over 100 Easy and Delicious Recipes to
Burn Fat, Lose Weight, Get Lean and Feel Great!

First published in 2016 by Erin Rose Publishing

Text and illustration copyright © 2016 Erin Rose Publishing

ISBN: 978-0-9933204-5-3

A CIP record for this book is available from the British Library.

DISCLAIMER:

This book is not affiliated with the official Sirt Food Diet book, and is for informational purposes only and not intended as a substitute for the medical advice, diagnosis or treatment of a physician or qualified healthcare provider.

Although every care has been taken in compiling the recipes in this book we cannot accept responsibility for any problems which arise as a result of preparing one of the recipes. The author and publisher disclaim responsibility for any adverse effects that may arise from the use or application of the recipes in this book.

Contents

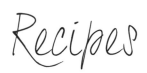

SNACKS

DRESSINGS

INTRODUCTION

This book is the perfect companion to the official SIRTfood Diet book and provides you with over 100 easy and delicious recipes rich in Sirt foods to make your SIRT Food Diet meal planning a breeze.

As you will have discovered if you have already read the official research, the SIRT Food Diet is all about incorporating a selection of sirtuin-activating 'wonder foods' into your diet to activate your fat-burning and muscle building genes! And the great news is that those super sirtuin-boosting foods include some delicious options: red wine, coffee, olive oil, rocket (arugula), dark chocolate, kale, strawberries and lots more!

The Sirt Food Diet is not a diet in the traditional sense of the word because it doesn't have to involve food restriction, it's more of a way of eating that aims to improve your overall health and promote weight loss.

Consuming foods rich in sirtuin-activating compounds has been shown to aid weight loss and help build additional lean muscle, which in turn boosts your metabolism, so jump start your fat-burning genes today with these easy and delicious Sirt food recipes!

In this book we have provided you with over 100 fantastic recipes, each of which contain as many Sirt foods as possible to maximise your intake.

In addition, each recipe has been calorie counted, so if you are looking to maximise weight-loss by reducing calories on some days, or combining the health benefits of Sirt foods with elements of intermittent fasting, you will be armed with the calorie count for each recipe and meal!

Plus, we have exciting ways to incorporate Sirt foods into your diet so you can still make lovely meals and delicious snacks — even those with an aversion to kale will enjoy our delicious pizza-style kale!

WHAT ARE THE SIRT FOODS?

There are many sirtuin-activating foods to choose from, with some containing more sirtuin-activating ingredients than others. These we have called the 'Top Sirt Foods' and these foods are included in all of our recipes, to maximise your Sirt food intake.

TOP SIRT FOODS

Buckwheat	Rocket (arugula)
Capers	Soy & Tofu products
Celery	Strawberries
Chicory (red)	Medjool dates
Chilli (bird's eye variety)	Turmeric (ground)
Cocoa	Walnuts
Coffee	Green tea
Kale	Red wine
Onion (red)	Olives and olive oil
Parsley	

OTHER SIRT FOODS

FRUITS

Blackberries

Blackcurrants

Blueberries

Apples

Cranberries

Goji berries

Grapes (red)

Plums

Raspberries

VEGETABLES

Artichokes

Asparagus

Broccoli

Chicory (yellow)

Endive lettuce

Green beans

Pak choi (bok choy)

Onions (white)

Shallots

Watercress

OTHER

Chestnuts	Quinoa
Chia seeds	Wholemeal flour
Peanuts	Ginger
Pistachios	Chilli peppers
Sunflower seeds	Chives
Cannellini beans	Dill
Haricot beans	Peppermint
Broad beans	Oregano
Corn (popcorn)	Sage

COOKING WITH SIRT FOODS

Now that you have read the list of Sirt foods it's time to plan your menu so that you can shop for all your required ingredients. If possible, aim to buy your fresh ingredients every few days and include Sirt foods in every meal.

By far the best way to load up on those Sirt foods is to start your day with a healthy smoothie. Especially a green one as it's a great refreshing kick start to your body and you can easily pack in 5 fruits/vegetables in one drink. It's sure to keep hunger away too!

We've provided lots of recipes for smoothies which you can not only have for breakfast but as a lunch replacement or mid-day snack. Bear in mind that although the recipes have been categorised as breakfast, light bites and main meals etc. you are free to swap them around.

If you have had a busy day and haven't been able to pack in the Sirt goodies as much as you would like, you can always supplement with a handful of walnuts, a green tea or a coffee in between meals to give you a boost and keep hunger away.

If you are being careful with your calorie intake you can be guided by the information on each recipe. A little word of caution when it comes to dates or 'nature's toffees' as some people call them – they are rich in calories. One date contains around 61 calories, so don't go overboard. That said, if you would normally reach for cakes, sweets or biscuits then a date or two is a good substitute because you won't be consuming empty refined sugar calories, but you'll still be enjoying a sweet treat.

If you haven't already, swap your normal cuppa for green tea which has virtually zero calories. If you don't have a taste for it you can try it with a flavouring such as jasmine, or even try the recipe for iced cranberry green tea for a refreshing way to drink it. Matcha, which is a type of green tea, is an even more powerful tea which also comes in a powder which can be added to smoothies and cooking. Health shops stock matcha, or alternatively, you can buy it online.

Keep a parsley plant on your window ledge because you can add it to virtually anything or even nibble on a sprig! Lovage is a relative of parsley which has even greater sirtuin-activating benefits, so if you can find it (and it's a big IF) use that instead of parsley. Because it's not so easy to find, we have not included lovage in any of these recipes, but if you do get hold of some just add it in.

Capers are available in most supermarkets and sold in jars. They do have a strong salty flavour so you won't need to use too many.

When it comes to chocolate, don't be tempted to buy a sugar-laden milk chocolate bar at the check-out because it won't contain much cocoa. Always aim for good quality dark chocolate with a high cocoa content of around 85% cocoa. Yes, it is more bitter, but your taste buds will soon adapt, and a square of chocolate after a meal is a great treat to round off the day.

Enjoy the recipes!

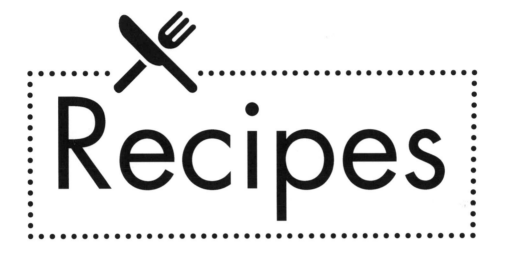

Recipes

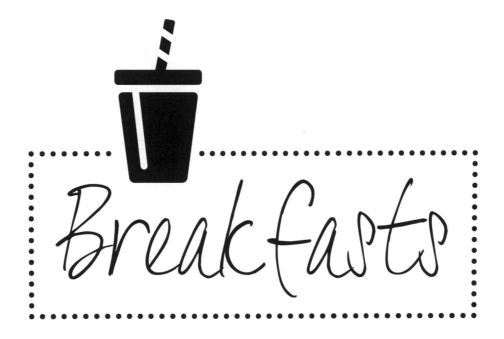

Breakfasts

Sirt Food Cocktail

Ingredients

75g (3oz) kale
50g (2oz) strawberries
1 apple, cored
2 sticks of celery
1 tablespoon parsley
1 teaspoon of matcha powder
Squeeze lemon juice (optional) to taste

Serves 1
101 calories per serving

Method

Place the ingredients into a blender and add enough water to cover the ingredients and blitz to a smooth consistency.

Summer Berry Smoothie

Ingredients

50g (2oz) blueberries
50g (2oz) strawberries
25g (1oz) blackcurrants
25g (1oz) red grapes
1 carrot, peeled
1 orange, peeled
Juice of 1 lime

Serves 1
146 calories per serving

Method

Place all of the ingredients into a blender and cover them with water. Blitz until smooth. You can also add some crushed ice and a mint leaf to garnish.

Mango, Celery & Ginger Smoothie

Ingredients

1 stalk of celery

50g (2oz) kale

1 apple, cored

50g (2oz) mango, peeled, de-stoned
and chopped

2.5cm (1 inch) chunk of fresh ginger root,
peeled and chopped

Method

Put all the ingredients into a blender with some water, and blitz until smooth.
Add ice to make your smoothie really refreshing.

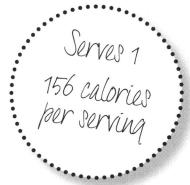

Serves 1
105 calories
per serving

Orange, Carrot & Kale Smoothie

Ingredients

1 carrot, peeled

1 orange, peeled

1 stick of celery

1 apple, cored

50g (2oz) kale

½ teaspoon matcha powder

Method

Place all of the ingredients into a blender and add in enough water to cover them.
Process until smooth, serve and enjoy.

Serves 1
156 calories
per serving

Creamy Strawberry & Cherry Smoothie

Ingredients

100g (3½ oz) strawberries

75g (3oz) frozen pitted cherries

1 tablespoon plain full-fat yogurt

175mls (6fl oz) unsweetened soya milk

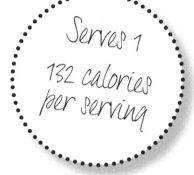

*Serves 1
132 calories per serving*

Method

Place all of the ingredients into a blender and process until smooth. Serve and enjoy.

Grape, Celery & Parsley Reviver

Ingredients

75g (3oz) red grapes

3 sticks of celery

1 avocado, de-stoned and peeled

1 tablespoon fresh parsley

½ teaspoon matcha powder

*Serves 1
134 calories per serving*

Method

Place all of the ingredients into a blender with enough water to cover them and blitz until smooth and creamy. Add crushed ice to make it even more refreshing.

Strawberry & Citrus Blend

Ingredients

75g (3oz) strawberries

1 apple, cored

1 orange, peeled

½ avocado, peeled and de-stoned

½ teaspoon matcha powder

Juice of 1 lime

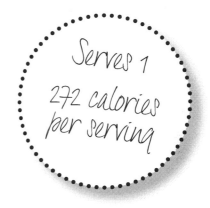

Serves 1
272 calories per serving

Method

Place all of the ingredients into a blender with enough water to cover them and process until smooth.

Grapefruit & Celery Blast

Ingredients

1 grapefruit, peeled

2 stalks of celery

50g (2oz) kale

½ teaspoon matcha powder

Serves 1
71 calories per serving

Method

Place all the ingredients into a blender with enough water to cover them and blitz until smooth.

Orange & Celery Crush

Ingredients

1 carrot, peeled

3 stalks of celery

1 orange, peeled

½ teaspoon matcha powder

Juice of 1 lime

Serves 1
95 calories per serving

Method

Place all of the ingredients into a blender with enough water to cover them and blitz until smooth.

Tropical Chocolate Delight

Ingredients

1 mango, peeled & de-stoned

75g (3oz) fresh pineapple, chopped

50g (2oz) kale

25g (1oz) rocket

1 tablespoon 100% cocoa powder or cacao nibs

150mls (5fl oz) coconut milk

Serves 1
427 calories per serving

Method

Place all of the ingredients into a blender and blitz until smooth. You can add a little water if it seems too thick.

Walnut & Spiced Apple Tonic

Ingredients

6 walnuts halves

1 apple, cored

1 banana

½ teaspoon matcha powder

½ teaspoon cinnamon

Pinch of ground nutmeg

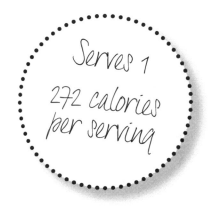

Serves 1
272 calories
per serving

Method

Place all of the ingredients into a blender and add sufficient water to cover them. Blitz until smooth and creamy.

Pineapple & Cucumber Smoothie

Ingredients

50g (2oz) cucumber

1 stalk of celery

2 slices of fresh pineapple

2 sprigs of parsley

½ teaspoon matcha powder

Squeeze of lemon juice

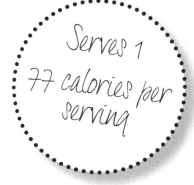

Serves 1
77 calories per
serving

Method

Place all of the ingredients into blender with enough water to cover them and blitz until smooth.

Sweet Rocket (Arugula) Boost

Ingredients

25g (1oz) fresh rocket (arugula) leaves

75g (3oz) kale

1 apple

1 carrot

1 tablespoon fresh parsley

Juice of 1 lime

Serves 1
113 calories per serving

Method

Place all of the ingredients into a blender with enough water to cover and process until smooth.

Avocado, Celery & Pineapple Smoothie

Ingredients

50g (2oz) fresh pineapple, peeled and chopped

3 stalks of celery

1 avocado, peeled & de-stoned

1 teaspoon fresh parsley

½ teaspoon matcha powder

Juice of ½ lemon

Serves 1
306 calories per serving

Method

Place all of the ingredients into a blender and add enough water to cover them. Process until creamy and smooth.

Banana & Ginger Snap

Ingredients

2.5cm (1 inch) chunk of fresh ginger, peeled

1 banana

1 large carrot

1 apple, cored

½ stick of celery

¼ level teaspoon turmeric powder

Serves 1
166 calories
per serving

Method

Place all the ingredients into a blender with just enough water to cover them.
Process until smooth

Chocolate, Strawberry & Coconut Crush

Ingredients

100mls (3½fl oz) coconut milk

100g (3½ oz) strawberries

1 banana

1 tablespoon 100% cocoa powder or cacao nibs

1 teaspoon matcha powder

Serves 1
324 calories per serving

Method

Toss all of the ingredients into a blender and process them to a creamy
consistency. Add a little extra water if you need to thin it a little.

Chocolate Berry Blend

Ingredients

50g (2oz) kale

50g (2oz) blueberries

50g (2oz) strawberries

1 banana

1 tablespoon 100% cocoa powder or cacao nibs

200mls (7fl oz) unsweetened soya milk

*Serves 1
241 calories per serving*

Method

Place all of the ingredients into a blender with enough water to cover them and process until smooth.

Cranberry & Kale Crush

Ingredients

75g (3oz) strawberries

50g (2oz) kale

120mls (4fl oz) unsweetened cranberry juice

1 teaspoon chia seeds

½ teaspoon matcha powder

*Serves 1
71 calories per serving*

Method

Place all of the ingredients into a blender and process until smooth. Add some crushed ice and a mint leaf or two for a really refreshing drink.

Mango & Rocket (Arugula) Smoothie

Ingredients

25g (1oz) fresh rocket (arugula)

150g (5oz) fresh mango, peeled, de-stoned and chopped

1 avocado, de-stoned and peeled

½ teaspoon matcha powder

Juice of 1 lime

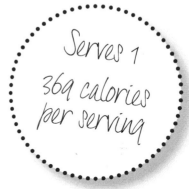

Serves 1
369 calories per serving

Method

Place all of the ingredients into a blender with enough water to cover them and process until smooth. Add a few ice cubes and enjoy.

Poached Eggs & Rocket (Arugula)

Ingredients

2 eggs

25g (1oz) fresh rocket (arugula)

1 teaspoon olive oil

Sea salt

Freshly ground black pepper

Serves 1
178 calories per serving

Method

Scatter the rocket (arugula) leaves onto a plate and drizzle the olive oil over them. Bring a shallow pan of water to the boil, add in the eggs and cook until the whites become firm. Serve the eggs on top of the rocket and season with salt and pepper.

Strawberry Buckwheat Pancakes

Ingredients

100g (3½oz) strawberries, chopped

100g (3½oz) buckwheat flour

1 egg

250mls (8fl oz) milk

1 teaspoon olive oil

1 teaspoon olive oil for frying

Freshly squeezed juice of 1 orange

*Makes 4
175 calories
per serving*

Method

Pour the milk into a bowl and mix in the egg and a teaspoon of olive oil. Sift in the flour to the liquid mixture until smooth and creamy. Allow it to rest for 15 minutes. Heat a little oil in a pan and pour in a quarter of the mixture (or to the size you prefer.) Sprinkle in a quarter of the strawberries into the batter. Cook for around 2 minutes on each side. Serve hot with a drizzle of orange juice. You could try experimenting with other berries such as blueberries and blackberries.

Strawberry & Nut Granola

Ingredients

200g (7oz) oats

250g (9oz) buckwheat flakes

100g (3½oz) walnuts, chopped

100g (3½oz) almonds, chopped

100g (3½oz) dried strawberries

1½ teaspoons ground ginger

1½ teaspoons ground cinnamon

120mls (4fl oz) olive oil

2 tablespoons honey

Serves 1
391 calories
per serving

Method

Combine the oats, buckwheat flakes, nuts, ginger and cinnamon. In a saucepan, warm the oil and honey. Stir until the honey has melted. Pour the warm oil into the dry ingredients and mix well. Spread the mixture out on a large baking tray (or two) and bake in the oven at 150C (300F) for around 50 minutes until the granola is golden. Allow it to cool. Add in the dried berries. Store in an airtight container until ready to use. Can be served with yogurt, milk or even dry as a handy snack.

Chilled Strawberry & Walnut Porridge

Ingredients

100g (3½oz) strawberries

50g (2oz) rolled oats

4 walnut halves, chopped

1 teaspoon chia seeds

200mls (7fl oz) unsweetened soya milk

100mls (3½ fl oz) water

*Sereves 1
384 calories per serving*

Method

Place the strawberries, oats, soya milk and water into a blender and process until smooth. Stir in the chia seeds and mix well. Chill in the fridge overnight and serve in the morning with a sprinkling of chopped walnuts. It's simple and delicious.

Fruit & Nut Yogurt Crunch

Ingredients

100g (3½ oz) plain Greek yogurt

50g (2oz) strawberries, chopped

6 walnut halves, chopped

Sprinkling of cocoa powder

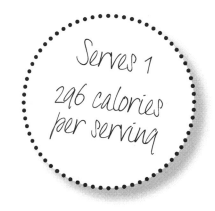

Serves 1
296 calories
per serving

Method

Stir half of the chopped strawberries into the yogurt. Using a glass, place a layer of yogurt with a sprinkling of strawberries and walnuts, followed by another layer of the same until you reach the top of the glass. Garnish with walnuts pieces and a dusting of cocoa powder.

Cheesy Baked Eggs

Ingredients

4 large eggs

75g (3oz) cheese, grated

25g (1oz) fresh rocket (arugula) leaves, finely chopped

1 tablespoon parsley

½ teaspoon ground turmeric

1 tablespoon olive oil

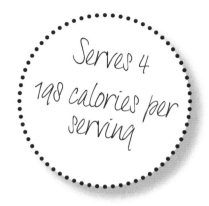

*Serves 4
198 calories per serving*

Method

Grease each ramekin dish with a little olive oil. Divide the rocket (arugula) between the ramekin dishes then break an egg into each one. Sprinkle a little parsley and turmeric on top then sprinkle on the cheese. Place the ramekins in a preheated oven at 220C/425F for 15 minutes, until the eggs are set and the cheese is bubbling.

Green Egg Scramble

Ingredients

2 eggs, whisked

25g (1oz) rocket (arugula) leaves

1 teaspoon chives, chopped

1 teaspoon fresh basil, chopped

1 teaspoon fresh parsley, chopped

1 tablespoon olive oil

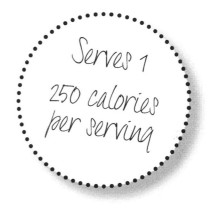

Serves 1
250 calories
per serving

Method

Mix the eggs together with the rocket (arugula) and herbs. Heat the oil in a frying pan and pour into the egg mixture. Gently stir until it's lightly scrambled. Season and serve.

Spiced Scramble

Ingredients

25g (1oz) kale, finely chopped

2 eggs

1 spring onion (scallion) finely chopped

1 teaspoon turmeric

1 tablespoon olive oil

Sea salt

Freshly ground black pepper

*Serves 1
259 calories
per serving*

Method

Crack the eggs into a bowl. Add the turmeric and whisk them. Season with salt and pepper. Heat the oil in a frying pan, add the kale and spring onion (scallion) and cook until it has wilted. Pour in the beaten eggs and stir until eggs have scrambled together with the kale.

Light Bites

Olive, Tomato & Herb Frittata

Ingredients

50g (2oz) Cheddar cheese, grated (shredded)

75g (3oz) pitted black olives, halved

8 cherry tomatoes, halved

4 large eggs

1 tablespoon fresh parsley, chopped

1 teaspoon fresh basil, chopped

1 tablespoon olive oil

Serves 2
381 calories per serving

Method

Break the eggs into a bowl and whisk them then add in the parsley, basil, olives and tomatoes. Add in the cheese and stir it. Heat the oil in a small frying pan land pour in the egg mixture. Cook until the egg mixture completely sets. Place the frittata under a hot grill for 3 minutes to finish it off. Carefully remove it from the pan. Cut into slices and serve.

Mushroom & Red Onion Buckwheat Pancakes

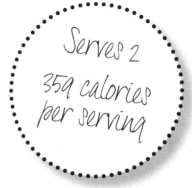

Serves 2
359 calories per serving

Ingredients

For the pancakes:

125g (4oz) buckwheat flour

1 egg

150mls (5fl oz) semi-skimmed milk

150mls (5fl oz) water

1 teaspoon olive oil for frying

For the filling:

1 red onion, chopped

75g (3½ oz) mushrooms, sliced

50g (2oz) spinach leaves

1 tablespoon fresh parsley, chopped

1 teaspoon olive oil

50g (2oz) rocket (arugula) leaves

Method

Sift the flour into a bowl and mix in an egg. Pour in the milk and water and mix to a smooth batter. Set aside. Heat a teaspoon of olive oil in a pan. Add the onion and mushrooms and cook for 5 minutes. Add the spinach and allow it to wilt. Set aside and keep it warm. Heat a teaspoon of oil in a frying pan and pour in half of the batter. Cook for 2 minutes on each side until golden. Spoon the spinach and mushroom mixture onto the pancake and add the parsley. Fold it over and serve onto a scattering of rocket (arugula) leaves. Repeat for the remaining mixture.

Kale & Feta Salad With Cranberry Dressing

Ingredients

250g (9oz) kale, finely chopped

50g (2oz) walnuts, chopped

75g (3oz) feta cheese, crumbled

1 apple, peeled, cored and sliced

4 medjool dates, chopped

For the Dressing

75g (3oz) cranberries

½ red onion, chopped

3 tablespoons olive oil

3 tablespoons water

2 teaspoons honey

1 tablespoon red wine vinegar

Sea salt

Serves 4
342 calories per serving

Method

Place the ingredients for the dressing into a food processor and process until smooth. If it seems too thick you can add a little extra water if necessary. Place all the ingredients for the salad into a bowl. Pour on the dressing and toss the salad until it is well coated in the mixture.

Tuna, Egg & Caper Salad

Ingredients

100g (3½oz) red chicory (or yellow if not available)

150g (5oz) tinned tuna flakes in brine, drained

100g (3 ½ oz) cucumber

25g (1oz) rocket (arugula)

6 pitted black olives

2 hard-boiled eggs, peeled and quartered

2 tomatoes, chopped

2 tablespoons fresh parsley, chopped

1 red onion, chopped

1 stalk of celery

1 tablespoon capers

2 tablespoons garlic vinaigrette (see recipe)

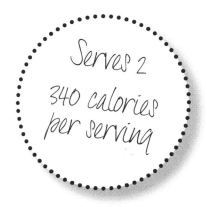

Serves 2
340 calories
per serving

Method

Place the tuna, cucumber, olives, tomatoes, onion, chicory, celery, parsley and rocket (arugula) into a bowl. Pour in the vinaigrette and toss the salad in the dressing. Serve onto plates and scatter the eggs and capers on top.

Hot Chicory & Nut Salad

Ingredients

For the salad:

100g (3½oz) green beans

100g (3½oz) red chicory, chopped (if unavailable use yellow chicory)

100g (3½oz) celery, chopped

25g (1oz) macadamia nuts, chopped

25g (1oz) walnuts, chopped

25g (1oz) plain peanuts, chopped

2 tomatoes, chopped

1 tablespoon olive oil

For the dressing:

2 tablespoons fresh parsley, finely chopped

½ teaspoon turmeric

½ teaspoon mustard

1 tablespoon olive oil

25mls (1fl oz) red wine vinegar

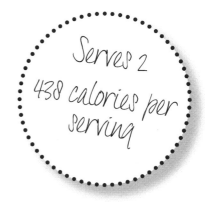

Serves 2
438 calories per serving

Method

Mix together the ingredients for the dressing then set them aside. Heat a tablespoon of olive oil in a frying pan then add the green beans, chicory and celery. Cook until the vegetables have softened then add in the chopped tomatoes and cook for 2 minutes. Add the prepared dressing, and thoroughly coat all of the vegetables. Serve onto plates and sprinkle the mixture of nuts over the top. Eat immediately.

Honey Chilli Squash

Ingredients

2 red onions, roughly chopped

2.5cm (1 inch) chunk of ginger root, finely chopped

2 cloves of garlic

2 bird's-eye chillies, finely chopped

1 butternut squash, peeled and chopped

100mls (3½ fl oz) vegetable stock (broth)

1 tablespoon olive oil

Juice of 1 orange

Juice of 1 limes

2 teaspoons honey

*Serves 4
118 calories per serving*

Method

Warm the oil in a pan and add in the red onions, squash chunks, chillies, garlic, ginger and honey. Cook for 3 minutes. Squeeze in the lime and orange juice. Pour in the stock (broth), orange and lime juice and cook for 15 minutes until tender.

Serrano Ham & Rocket (Arugula)

Ingredients

175g (6oz) Serrano ham

125g (4oz) rocket (arugula) leaves

2 tablespoons olive oil

1 tablespoon orange juice

Method

Pour the oil and juice into a bowl and toss the rocket (arugula) in the mixture. Serve the rocket onto plates and top it off with the ham.

Serves 4
159 calories per serving

Pasta Salad

Ingredients

275g (10oz) buckwheat pasta

225g (8oz) green beans

100g (3½ oz) cherry tomatoes

2 cloves of garlic, crushed

1 red onion, finely chopped

1 bird's-eye chilli, finely chopped

2 tablespoons smooth peanut butter

150mls (5fl oz) coconut milk

1 tablespoon tomato puree

½ teaspoon turmeric powder

2 tablespoons olive oil

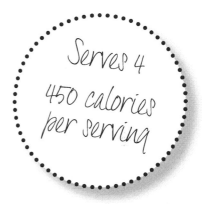

Serves 4
450 calories
per serving

Method

Cook the buckwheat according to the instructions, then set aside and keep warm.
Heat the olive oil in a large frying pan or wok. Add the garlic and onion and
cook for 1 minute. Add in the green beans and cook for 3 minutes. Add
in the tomatoes and cook for 2 minutes. In a separate bowl mix the peanut
butter, coconut milk, turmeric, tomato puree and chilli. Add the pasta and
coconut mixture to the vegetables. Stir well, making sure everything is well
coated. Serve alongside a leafy green salad.

Hot Chorizo, Tomato & Kale Salad

Ingredients

225g (8oz) kale leaves, finely chopped

75g (3oz) chorizo sausage, thinly sliced

8 cherry tomatoes

2 cloves of garlic

1 red onion, finely chopped

2 tablespoons olive oil

2 tablespoons red wine vinegar

Sea salt

Freshly ground black pepper

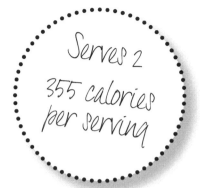

Serves 2
355 calories
per serving

Method

Heat the olive oil into a frying pan and add the sliced chorizo, garlic, onion and tomatoes. Cook for around 5 minutes. Add in the red wine vinegar and kale and cook for around 7 minutes or until the kale has softened. Season with salt and pepper. Serve immediately.

Red Chicory & Walnut Coleslaw

Ingredients

100g (3½ oz) red chicory, (or yellow) finely grated (shredded)

5 stalks of celery, finely chopped

8 walnut halves, chopped

1 red onion, finely chopped

2 tablespoons mayonnaise

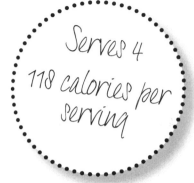

Serves 4
118 calories per serving

Method

Place all of the ingredients into a bowl and combine well. Chill in the fridge before serving.

Smoked Salmon & Chicory Boats

Ingredients

150g (5oz) red chicory leaves (or yellow if it's unavailable)

150g (5oz) smoked salmon, finely chopped

100g (3½oz) cucumber, diced

2 tablespoons fresh parsley, chopped

½ red onion, finely chopped

Juice of 1 lime

2 tablespoons olive oil

Serves 4
152 calories per serving

Method

Place the salmon, cucumber, onion, parsley, oil and lime juice into a bowl and toss the ingredients well. Scoop some of the salmon mixture into each of the chicory leaves and chill before serving.

Vegetable & Nut Loaf

Ingredients

175g (6oz) mushrooms, finely chopped

100g (3½ oz) haricot beans

100g (3½ oz) walnuts, finely chopped

100g (3½ oz) peanuts, finely chopped

1 carrot, finely chopped

3 sticks celery, finely chopped

1 bird's-eye chilli, finely chopped

1 red onion, finely chopped

1 egg, beaten

2 cloves of garlic, chopped

2 tablespoons olive oil

2 teaspoons turmeric powder

2 tablespoons soy sauce

4 tablespoons fresh parsley, chopped

100mls (3½ fl oz) water

60mls (2fl oz) red wine

*Serves 4
453 calories
per serving*

Method

Heat the oil in a pan and add the garlic, chilli, carrot, celery, onion, mushrooms and turmeric. Cook for 5 minutes. Place the haricot beans in a bowl and stir in the nuts, vegetables, soy sauce, egg, parsley, red wine and water. Grease and line a large loaf tin with greaseproof paper. Spoon the mixture into the loaf tin, cover with foil and bake in the oven at 190C/375F for 60-90 minutes. Let it stand for 10 minutes then turn onto a serving plate.

Dates & Parma Ham

Ingredients

12 medjool dates

2 slices of Parma ham, cut into strips

Method

Wrap each date with a strip of Parma ham. Can be served hot or cold.

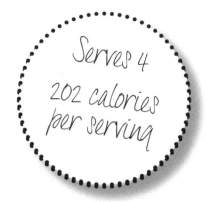

Serves 4
202 calories per serving

Braised Celery

Ingredients

250g (9oz) celery, chopped

100mls (3½ fl oz) warm vegetable stock (broth)

1 red onion, chopped

1 clove of garlic, crushed

1 tablespoon fresh parsley, chopped

25g (1oz) butter

Sea salt and freshly ground black pepper

Serves 4
67 calories per serving

Method

Place the celery, onion, stock (broth) and garlic into a saucepan and bring it to the boil, reduce the heat and simmer for 10 minutes. Stir in the parsley and butter and season with salt and pepper. Serve as an accompaniment to roast meat dishes.

Cheesy Buckwheat Cakes

Ingredients

100g (3½oz) buckwheat, cooked and cooled

1 large egg

25g (1oz) cheddar cheese, grated (shredded)

25g (1oz) wholemeal breadcrumbs

2 shallots, chopped

2 tablespoons fresh parsley, chopped

1 tablespoon olive oil

Serves 2
358 calories per serving

Method

Crack the egg into a bowl, whisk it then set aside. In a separate bowl combine all the buckwheat, cheese, shallots and parsley and mix well. Pour in the beaten egg to the buckwheat mixture and stir well. Shape the mixture into patties. Scatter the breadcrumbs on a plate and roll the patties in them. Heat the olive oil in a large frying pan and gently place the cakes in the oil. Cook for 3-4 minutes on either side until slightly golden.

Red Chicory & Stilton Cheese Boats

Ingredients

200g (7oz) stilton cheese, crumbled

200g (7oz) red chicory leaves (or if unavailable, use yellow)

2 tablespoons fresh parsley, chopped

1 tablespoon olive oil

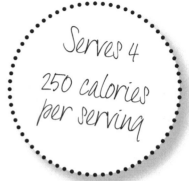

Serves 4
250 calories per serving

Method

Place the red chicory leaves onto a baking sheet. Drizzle them with olive oil then sprinkle the cheese inside the leaves. Place them under a hot grill (broiler) for around 4 minutes until the cheese has melted. Sprinkle with chopped parsley and serve straight away.

Strawberry, Rocket (Arugula) & Feta Salad

Ingredients

75g (3oz) fresh rocket (arugula) leaves

75g (3oz) feta cheese, crumbled

100g (3½ oz) strawberries, halved

8 walnut halves

2 tablespoons flaxseeds

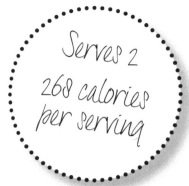

Serves 2
268 calories
per serving

Method

Combine all the ingredients in a bowl then scatter them onto two plates. For an extra sirt food boost you can drizzle over some olive oil.

Mushroom Courgetti & Lemon Caper Pesto

Ingredients

4 courgettes (zucchinis)

10 oyster mushrooms, sliced

1 red onion, sliced

2 tablespoons olive oil

2 tablespoons lemon caper pesto (see recipe)

50g (2oz) rocket (arugula) leaves

Serves 4
127 calories per serving

Method

Spiralize the courgettes into spaghetti. If you don't have a spiralizer, finely cut the vegetables lengthways into long 'spaghetti' strips. Heat the olive oil in a frying pan, add the mushrooms and onions and cook for minutes. Add in the courgettes and the pesto and cook for 5 minutes. Scatter the rocket (arugula) leaves onto plates and serve the courgettes on top.

Chicken Stir-Fry

Ingredients

150g (5oz) egg noodles

50g (2oz) cauliflower florets, roughly chopped

25g (1oz) kale, finely chopped

25g (1oz) mange tout

2 sticks of celery, finely chopped

2 chicken breasts

1 red pepper (bell pepper), chopped

1 clove of garlic

2 tablespoons soy sauce

100mls (3½ fl oz) chicken stock (broth)

1 tablespoon olive oil

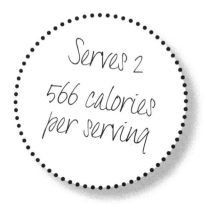

Serves 2
566 calories
per serving

Method

Cook the noodles according to the instructions then set aside and keep warm. Heat the oil in a wok or frying pan and add in the garlic and chicken. Add in the kale, celery, cauliflower, red pepper (bell pepper), mange tout and cook for 4 minutes. Pour in the chicken stock (broth) and soy sauce and cook for 3 minutes or until the chicken is thoroughly cooked. Stir in the cooked noodles and serve.

Tuna With Lemon Herb Dressing

Ingredients

4 tuna steaks

1 tablespoon olive oil

For the dressing:

25g (1oz) pitted green olives, chopped

2 tablespoons fresh parsley, chopped

1 tablespoon fresh basil, chopped

2 tablespoons olive oil

Freshly squeezed juice of 1 lemon

Serves 4
241 calories per serving

Method

Heat a tablespoon of olive oil in a griddle pan. Add the tuna steaks and cook on a high heat for 2-3 minutes on each side. Reduce the cooking time if you want them rare. Place the ingredients for the dressing into a bowl and combine them well. Serve the tuna steaks with a dollop of dressing over them. Serve alongside a leafy rocket salad.

Kale, Apple & Fennel Soup

Ingredients

450g (1lb) kale, chopped

200g (7oz) fennel, chopped

2 apples, peeled, cored and chopped

2 tablespoons fresh parsley, chopped

1 tablespoon olive oil

Sea salt

Freshly ground black pepper

*Serves 4
99 calories per serving*

Method

Heat the oil in a saucepan, add the kale and fennel and cook for 5 minutes until the fennel has softened. Stir in the apples and parsley. Cover with hot water, bring it to the boil and simmer for 10 minutes. Using a hand blender or food processor blitz until the soup is smooth. Season with salt and pepper.

Lentil Soup

Ingredients

175g (6oz) red lentils

1 red onion, chopped

1 clove of garlic, chopped

2 sticks of celery, chopped

2 carrots, chopped

½ bird's-eye chilli

1 teaspoon ground cumin

1 teaspoon ground turmeric

1 teaspoon ground coriander (cilantro)

1200mls (2 pints) vegetable stock (broth)

2 tablespoons olive oil

Sea salt

Freshly ground black pepper

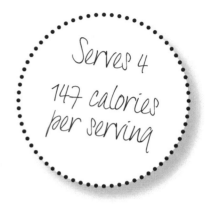

Serves 4
147 calories
per serving

Method

Heat the oil in a saucepan and add the onion and cook for 5 minutes. Add in the carrots, lentils, celery, chilli, coriander (cilantro), cumin, turmeric and garlic and cook for 5 minutes. Pour in the stock (broth), bring it to the boil, reduce the heat and simmer for 45 minutes. Using a hand blender or food processor, puree the soup until smooth. Season with salt and pepper. Serve.

Cauliflower & Walnut Soup

Ingredients

450g (1lb) cauliflower, chopped

8 walnut halves, chopped

1 red onion, chopped

900mls (1½ pints) vegetable stock (broth)

100mls (3½ fl oz) double cream (heavy cream)

½ teaspoon turmeric

1 tablespoon olive oil

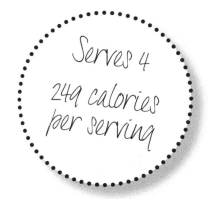

Serves 4
249 calories
per serving

Method

Heat the oil in a saucepan, add the cauliflower and red onion and cook for 4 minutes, stirring continuously. Pour in the stock (broth), bring to the boil and cook for 15 minutes. Stir in the walnuts, double cream and turmeric. Using a food processor or hand blender, process the soup until smooth and creamy. Serve into bowls and top off with a sprinkling of chopped walnuts.

Celery & Blue Cheese Soup

Ingredients

125g (4oz) blue cheese

25g (1oz) butter

1 head of celery (approx 650g)

1 red onion, chopped

900mls (1½ pints) chicken stock (broth)

150mls (5fl oz) single cream

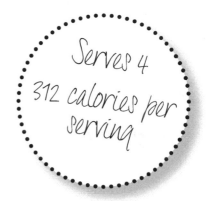

Serves 4
312 calories per serving

Method

Heat the butter in a saucepan, add the onion and celery and cook until the vegetables have softened. Pour in the stock, bring to the boil then reduce the heat and simmer for 15 minutes. Pour in the cream and stir in the cheese until it has melted. Serve and eat straight away.

Spicy Squash Soup

Ingredients

150g (5oz) kale

1 butternut squash, peeled, de-seeded and chopped

1 red onion, chopped

3 bird's-eye chillies, chopped

3 cloves of garlic

2 teaspoons turmeric

1 teaspoon ground ginger

600mls (1 pint) vegetable stock (broth)

2 tablespoons olive oil

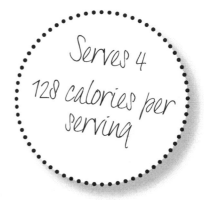

Serves 4
128 calories per serving

Method

Heat the olive oil in a saucepan, add the chopped butternut squash and onion and cook for 6 minutes until softened. Stir in the kale, garlic, chilli, turmeric and ginger and cook for 2 minutes, stirring constantly. Pour in the vegetable stock (broth) bring it to the boil and cook for 20 minutes. Using a blender process until smooth. Serve on its own or with a swirl of cream or crème fraiche. Enjoy.

French Onion Soup

Ingredients

750g (1¾lbs) red onions, thinly sliced

50g (2oz) Cheddar cheese, grated (shredded)

12g (½ oz) butter

2 teaspoons flour

2 slices wholemeal bread

1 litre (1½ pints) beef stock (broth)

1 tablespoon olive oil

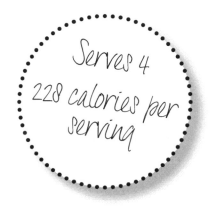

Serves 4
228 calories per serving

Method

Heat the butter and oil in a large pan. Add the onions and gently cook on a low heat for 25 minutes, stirring occasionally. Add in the flour and stir well. Pour in the stock (broth) and keep stirring. Bring to the boil, reduce the heat and simmer for 30 minutes. Cut the slices of bread into triangles, sprinkle with cheese and place them under a hot grill (broiler) until the cheese has melted. Serve the soup into bowls and add 2 triangles of cheesy toast on top. Enjoy.

Cream of Broccoli & Kale Soup

Ingredients

250g (9oz) broccoli

250g (9oz) kale

1 potato, peeled and chopped

1 red onion, chopped

600mls (1 pint) vegetable stock

300mls (½ pint) milk

1 tablespoon olive oil

Sea salt

Freshly ground black pepper

Serves 4
165 calories
per serving

Method

Heat the olive oil in a saucepan, add the onion and cook for 5 minutes. Add in the potato, kale and broccoli and cook for 5 minutes. Pour in the stock (broth) and milk and simmer for 20 minutes. Using a food processor or hand blender, process the soup until smooth and creamy. Season with salt and pepper.
Re-heat if necessary and serve.

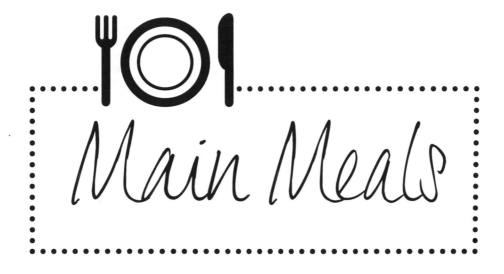

Main Meals

Coq Au Vin

Ingredients

450g (1lb) button mushrooms

100g (3½oz) streaky bacon, chopped

16 chicken thighs, skin removed

3 cloves of garlic, crushed

3 tablespoons fresh parsley, chopped

3 carrots, chopped

2 red onions, chopped

2 tablespoons plain flour

2 tablespoons olive oil

750mls (1¼ pints) red wine

1 bouquet garni

Serves 8
459 calories per serving

Method

Place the flour on a large plate and coat the chicken in it. Heat the olive oil in a large saucepan, add the chicken and brown it, before setting aside. Fry the bacon in the pan then add the onion and cook for 5 minutes. Pour in the red wine and add the chicken, carrots, bouquet garni and garlic. Transfer it to a large ovenproof dish. Cook in the oven at 180C/360F for 1 hour. Remove the bouquet garni and skim off any excess fat, if necessary. Add in the mushrooms and cook for 15 minutes. Stir in the parsley just before serving.

Turkey Satay Skewers

Ingredients

250g (9oz) turkey breast, cubed

25g (1oz) smooth peanut butter

1 clove of garlic, crushed

½ small bird's eye chilli (or more if you like it hotter), finely chopped

½ teaspoon ground turmeric

200mls (7fl oz) coconut milk

2 teaspoons soy sauce

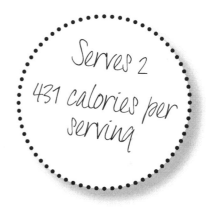

Serves 2
431 calories per serving

Method

Combine the coconut milk, peanut butter, turmeric, soy sauce, garlic and chilli. Add the turkey pieces to the bowl and stir them until they are completely coated. Push the turkey onto metal skewers. Place the satay skewers on a barbeque or under a hot grill (broiler) and cook for 4-5 minutes on each side, until they are completely cooked.

Salmon & Capers

Ingredients

75g (3oz) Greek yogurt

4 salmon fillets, skin removed

4 teaspoons Dijon Mustard

1 tablespoon capers, chopped

2 teaspoons fresh parsley

Zest of 1 lemon

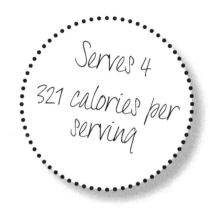

Serves 4
321 calories per serving

Method

In a bowl, mix together the yogurt, mustard, lemon zest, parsley and capers. Thoroughly coat the salmon in the mixture. Place the salmon under a hot grill (broiler) and cook for 3-4 minutes on each side, or until the fish is cooked. Serve with mashed potatoes and vegetables or a large green leafy salad.

Moroccan Chicken Casserole

Ingredients

250g (9oz) tinned chickpeas (garbanzo beans) drained

4 chicken breasts, cubed

4 medjool dates, halved

6 dried apricots, halved

1 red onion, sliced

1 carrot, chopped

1 teaspoon ground cumin

1 teaspoon ground cinnamon

1 teaspoon ground turmeric

1 bird's-eye chilli, chopped

600mls (1 pints) chicken stock (broth)

25g (1oz) cornflour

60mls (2fl oz) water

2 tablespoons fresh coriander (cilantro)

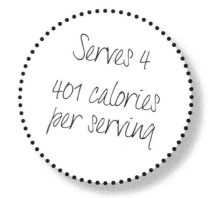

Serves 4
401 calories
per serving

Method

Place the chicken, chickpeas (garbanzo beans), onion, carrot, chilli, cumin, turmeric, cinnamon and stock (broth) into a large saucepan. Bring it to the boil, reduce the heat and simmer for 25 minutes. Add in the dates and apricots and simmer for 10 minutes. In a cup, mix the cornflour together with the water until it becomes a smooth paste. Pour the mixture into the saucepan and stir until it thickens. Add in the coriander (cilantro) and mix well. Serve with buckwheat or couscous.

Chilli Con Carne

Ingredients

450g (1lb) lean minced beef

400g (14oz) chopped tomatoes

200g (7oz) red kidney beans

2 tablespoons tomato purée

2 cloves of garlic, crushed

2 red onions, chopped

2 bird's-eye chillies, finely chopped

1 red pepper (bell pepper), chopped

1 stick of celery, finely chopped

1 tablespoon cumin

1 tablespoon turmeric

1 tablespoon cocoa powder

400mls (14 fl oz) beef stock (broth)

175mls (6fl oz) red wine

1 tablespoon olive oil

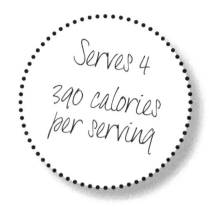

Serves 4
390 calories
per serving

Method

Heat the oil in a large saucepan, add the onion and cook for 5 minutes. Add in the garlic, celery, chilli, turmeric, and cumin and cook for 2 minutes before adding then meat then cook for another 5 minutes. Pour in the stock (broth), red wine, tomatoes, tomato purée, red pepper (bell pepper), kidney beans and cocoa powder. Simmer on a low heat for 45 minutes, keep it covered and stirring occasionally. Serve with brown rice or buckwheat.

Prawn & Coconut Curry

Ingredients

400g (14oz) tinned chopped tomatoes

400g (14oz) large prawns (shrimps), shelled and raw

25g (1oz) fresh coriander (cilantro) chopped

3 red onions, finely chopped

3 cloves of garlic, crushed

2 bird's-eye chillies

½ teaspoon ground coriander (cilantro)

½ teaspoon turmeric

400mls (14fl oz) coconut milk

1 tablespoons olive oil

Juice of 1 lime

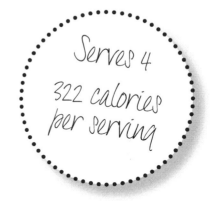

Serves 4
322 calories
per serving

Method

Place the onions, garlic, tomatoes, chillies, lime juice, turmeric, ground coriander (cilantro), chillies and half of the fresh coriander (cilantro) into a blender and blitz until you have a smooth curry paste. Heat the olive oil in a frying pan, add the paste and cook for 2 minutes. Stir in the coconut milk and warm it thoroughly. Add the prawns (shrimps) to the paste and cook them until they have turned pink and are completely cooked. Stir in the remaining fresh coriander (cilantro). Serve with rice.

Chicken & Bean Casserole

Ingredients

400g (14oz) chopped tomatoes

400g (14oz) tinned cannellini beans or haricot beans

8 chicken thighs, skin removed

2 carrots, peeled and finely chopped

2 red onions, chopped

4 sticks of celery

4 large mushrooms

2 red peppers (bell peppers), de-seeded and chopped

1 clove of garlic

2 tablespoons soy sauce

1 tablespoon olive oil

1.75 litres (3 pints) chicken stock (broth)

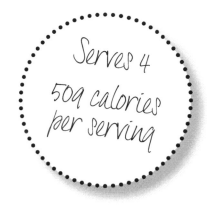

Serves 4
509 calories
per serving

Method

Heat the olive oil in a saucepan, add the garlic and onions and cook for 5 minutes. Add in the chicken and cook for 5 minutes then add the carrots, cannellini beans, celery, red peppers (bell peppers) and mushrooms. Pour in the stock (broth) soy sauce and tomatoes. Bring it to the boil, reduce the heat and simmer for 45 minutes. Serve with rice or new potatoes.

Mussels In Red Wine Sauce

Ingredients

800g (2lb) mussels

2 x 400g (14oz) tins of chopped tomatoes

25g (1oz) butter

1 tablespoon fresh chives, chopped

1 tablespoon fresh parsley, chopped

1 bird's-eye chilli, finely chopped

4 cloves of garlic, crushed

400mls (14fl oz) red wine

Juice of 1 lemon

Serves 2
364 calories
per serving

Method

Wash the mussels, remove their beards and set them aside. Heat the butter in a large saucepan and add in the red wine. Reduce the heat and add the parsley, chives, chilli and garlic whilst stirring. Add in the tomatoes, lemon juice and mussels. Cover the saucepan and cook for 3-4 minutes. Remove the saucepan from the heat and take out any mussels which haven't opened and discard them. Serve and eat immediately.

Roast Balsamic Vegetables

Ingredients

4 tomatoes, chopped

2 red onions, chopped

3 sweet potatoes, peeled and chopped

100g (3½oz) red chicory (or if unavailable, use yellow)

100g (3½ oz) kale, finely chopped

300g (11oz) potatoes, peeled and chopped

5 stalks of celery, chopped

1 bird's-eye chilli, de-seeded and finely chopped

2 tablespoons fresh parsley, chopped

2 tablespoons fresh coriander (cilantro) chopped

3 tablespoons olive oil

2 tablespoons balsamic vinegar

1 teaspoon mustard

Sea salt

Freshly ground black pepper

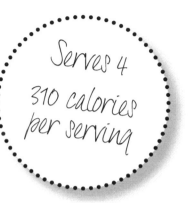

Serves 4
310 calories
per serving

Method

Place the olive oil, balsamic, mustard, parsley and coriander (cilantro) into a bowl and mix well. Toss all the remaining ingredients into the dressing and season with salt and pepper. Transfer the vegetables to an ovenproof dish and cook in the oven at 200C/400F for 45 minutes.

Tomato & Goat's Cheese Pizza

Ingredients

225g (8oz) buckwheat flour

2 teaspoons dried yeast

Pinch of salt

150mls (5fl oz) slightly warm water

1 teaspoon olive oil

For the Topping:

75g (3oz) feta cheese, crumbled

75g (3oz) passata (or tomato paste)

1 tomato, sliced

1 red onion, finely chopped

25g (1oz) rocket (arugula) leaves, chopped

Serves 2
562 calories
per serving

Method

In a bowl, combine all the ingredients for the pizza dough then allow it to stand for at least an hour until it has doubled in size. Roll the dough out to a size to suit you. Spoon the passata onto the base and add the rest of the toppings. Bake in the oven at 200C/400F for 15-20 minutes or until browned at the edges and crispy and serve.

Tofu Thai Curry

Ingredients

400g (14oz) tofu, diced

200g (7oz) sugar snap peas

5cm (2 inch) chunk fresh ginger root, peeled and finely chopped

2 red onions, chopped

2 cloves of garlic, crushed

2 bird's eye chillies

2 tablespoons tomato puree

1 stalk of lemon grass, inner stalks only

1 tablespoon fresh coriander (cilantro), chopped

1 teaspoon cumin

300mls (½ pint) coconut milk

200mls (7fl oz) vegetable stock (broth)

1 tablespoon virgin olive oil

Juice of 1 lime

Serves 4
270 calories per serving

Method

Heat the oil in a frying pan, add the onion and cook for 4 minutes. Add in the chillies, cumin, ginger, and garlic and cook for 2 minutes. Add the tomato puree, lemon grass, sugar-snap peas, lime juice and tofu and cook for 2 minutes. Pour in the stock (broth), coconut milk and coriander (cilantro) and simmer for 5 minutes. Serve with brown rice or buckwheat and a handful of rocket (arugula) leaves on the side.

Tender Spiced Lamb

Ingredients

1.35kg (3lb) lamb shoulder

3 red onions, sliced

3 cloves of garlic, crushed

1 bird's eye chilli, finely chopped

1 teaspoon turmeric

1 teaspoon ground cumin

½ teaspoon ground coriander (cilantro)

¼ teaspoon ground cinnamon

2 tablespoons olive oil

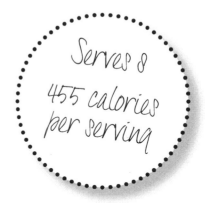

Serves 8
455 calories
per serving

Method

In a bowl, combine the chilli, garlic and spices with a tablespoon of olive oil. Coat the lamb with the spice mixture and marinate it for an hour, or overnight if you can. Heat the remaining oil in a pan, add the lamb and brown it for 3-4 minutes on all sides to seal it. Place the lamb in an ovenproof dish. Add in the red onions and cover the dish with foil. Transfer to the oven and roast at 170C/325F for 4 hours. The lamb should be extremely tender and falling off the bone. Serve with rice or couscous, salad or vegetables.

Chilli Cod Fillets

Ingredients

4 cod fillets (approx 150g each)

2 tablespoons fresh parsley, chopped

2 bird's-eye chillies (or more if you like it hot)

2 cloves of garlic, chopped

4 tablespoons olive oil

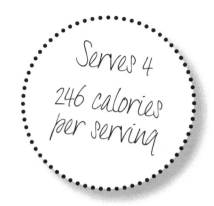

Serves 4
246 calories
per serving

Method

Heat a tablespoon of olive oil in a frying pan, add the fish and cook for 6-7 minutes or until thoroughly cooked, turning once halfway through. Remove and keep warm. Pour the remaining olive oil into the pan and add the chilli, chopped garlic and parsley. Warm it thoroughly. Serve the fish onto plates and pour the warm chilli oil over it.

Steak & Mushroom Noodles

Ingredients

100g (3½oz) shitake mushrooms, halved, if large

100g (3½oz) chestnut mushrooms, sliced

150g (5oz) udon noodles

75g (3oz) kale, finely chopped

75g (3oz) baby leaf spinach, chopped

2 sirloin steaks

2 tablespoons miso paste

2.5cm (1in) piece fresh ginger, finely chopped

2 tablespoons olive oil

1 star anise

1 red chilli, finely sliced

1 red onion, finely chopped

1 tablespoon fresh coriander (cilantro) chopped

1 litre (1½ pints) warm water

*Serves 4
296 calories
per serving*

Method

Pour the water into a saucepan and add in the miso, star anise and ginger. Bring it to the boil, reduce the heat and simmer gently. In the meantime, cook the noodles according to their instructions then drain them. Heat the oil in a saucepan, add the steak and cook for around 2-3 minutes on each side (or 1-2 minutes, for rare meat). Remove the meat and set aside. Place the mushrooms, spinach, coriander (cilantro) and kale into the miso broth and cook for 5 minutes. In the meantime, heat the remaining oil in a separate pan and fry the chilli and onion for 4 minutes, until softened. Serve the noodles into bowls and pour the soup on top. Thinly slice the steaks and add them to the top. Serve immediately.

Roast Lamb & Red Wine Sauce

Ingredients

1.5kg (3lb 6oz) leg of lamb

5 cloves of garlic

6 sprigs of rosemary

3 tablespoons parsley

1 tablespoon honey

1 tablespoon olive oil

½ teaspoon sea salt

300mls (½ pint) red wine

Serves 6
581 calories per serving

Method

Place the rosemary, garlic, parsley and salt into a pestle and mortar or small bowl and blend the ingredients together. Make small slits in the lamb and press a little of the mixture into each incision. Pour the oil over the meat and cover it with foil. Roast in the oven for around 1 hour 20 minutes.

Pour the wine into a small saucepan and stir in the honey. Warm the liquid then reduce the heat and simmer until reduced. Once the lamb is ready, pour the sauce over it, then return it to the oven to cook for another 5 minutes.

Cannellini & Spinach Curry

Ingredients

400g (14oz) cannellini beans

400g (14oz) tinned tomatoes

150g (5oz) cauliflower florets

75g (3oz) spinach

1 red onion, chopped

1 carrot, chopped

3 cloves of garlic, chopped

1 teaspoon ground cumin

1½ teaspoons turmeric

1 teaspoon curry powder

1 bird's-eye chilli, finely chopped

600mls (1 pint) vegetable stock (broth)

2 tablespoons olive oil

Serves 4
232 calories per serving

Method

Heat the oil in a saucepan. Add the onion, cauliflower, carrots and garlic and cook for 5 minutes until the vegetables soften. Add the cumin, turmeric, curry powder and chilli and stir for 2 minutes. Add the tomatoes, cannellini beans and stock (broth). Bring to the boil, reduce the heat and simmer for 25-30 minutes. Stir in the spinach for the last two minutes of cooking, until it has wilted. Serve with brown rice.

Turkey Curry

Ingredients

450g (1lb) turkey breasts, chopped

100g (3½ oz) fresh rocket (arugula) leaves

5 cloves garlic, chopped

3 teaspoons medium curry powder

2 teaspoons turmeric powder

2 tablespoons fresh coriander (cilantro), finely chopped

2 bird's-eye chillies, chopped

2 red onions, chopped

400mls (14fl oz) full-fat coconut milk

2 tablespoons olive oil

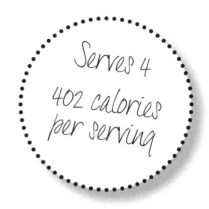

Serves 4
402 calories
per serving

Method

Heat the olive oil in a saucepan, add the chopped red onions and cook them for around 5 minutes or until soft. Stir in the garlic and the turkey and cook it for 7-8 minutes. Stir in the turmeric, chillies and curry powder then add the coconut milk and coriander (cilantro). Bring it to the boil, reduce the heat and simmer for around 10 minutes. Scatter the rocket (arugula) onto plates and spoon the curry on top. Serve alongside brown rice.

Chilli Tomato King Prawns

Ingredients

100g (3½oz) pak choi (bok choy)

24 raw king prawns (jumbo shrimp), shelled

4 tomatoes, chopped

2 bird's eye chillies, chopped

1 tablespoon fresh coriander (cilantro), chopped

1 tablespoon fresh parsley, chopped

2 tablespoons olive oil

*Serves 4
121 calories per serving*

Method

Heat a tablespoon of oil in a frying pan and add in the prawns (shrimps) and cook until they are completely pink. Remove and set aside. Heat another tablespoon of oil in a pan and add the pak choi (bok choy), tomatoes and chilli peppers. Cook for 3 minutes. Return the prawns to the pan and warm through. Sprinkle with chopped parsley and coriander (cilantro) and stir. Serve with brown rice and salad.

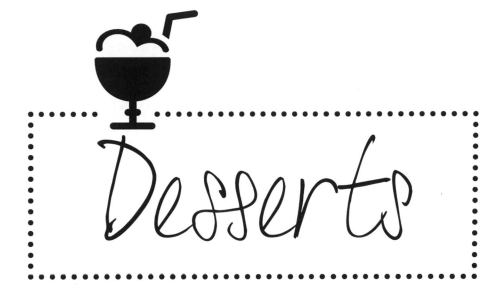

Desserts

Fruit Skewers & Strawberry Dip

Ingredients

150g (5oz) red grapes

1 pineapple, (approx 2lb weight) peeled and diced

400g (14oz) strawberries

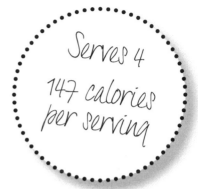

Serves 4
147 calories
per serving

Method

Place 100g (3½ oz) of the strawberries into a food processor and blend until smooth. Pour the dip into a serving bowl. Skewer the grapes, pineapple chunks and remaining strawberries onto skewers. Serve alongside the strawberry dip.

Chocolate Nut Truffles

Ingredients

150g (5oz) desiccated (shredded) coconut

50g (2oz) walnuts, chopped

25g (1oz) hazelnuts, chopped

4 medjool dates

2 tablespoons 100% cocoa powder or cacao nibs

1 tablespoon coconut oil

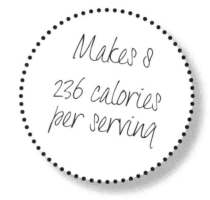

Makes 8
236 calories
per serving

Method

Place all of the ingredients into a blender and process until smooth and creamy. Using a teaspoon, scoop the mixture into bite-size pieces then roll it into balls. Place them into small paper cases, cover them and chill for 1 hour before serving.

No-Bake Strawberry Flapjacks

Ingredients

75g (3oz) porridge oats

125g (4oz) dates

50g (2oz) strawberries

50g (2oz) peanuts (unsalted)

50g (2oz) walnuts

1 tablespoon coconut oil

2 tablespoons 100% cocoa powder or cacao nibs

Makes 8
182 calories per serving

Method

Place all of the ingredients into a blender and process until they become a soft consistency. Spread the mixture onto a baking sheet or small flat tin. Press the mixture down and smooth it out. Cut it into 8 pieces, ready to serve. You can add an extra sprinkling of cocoa powder to garnish if you wish.

Chocolate Balls

Ingredients

50g (2oz) peanut butter (or almond butter)

25g (1oz) cocoa powder

25g (1oz) desiccated (shredded) coconut

1 tablespoon honey

1 tablespoon cocoa powder for coating

Method

Place the ingredients into a bowl and mix. Using a teaspoon scoop out a little of the mixture and shape it into a ball. Roll the ball in a little cocoa powder and set aside. Repeat for the remaining mixture. Can be eaten straight away or stored in the fridge.

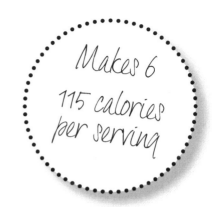

Makes 6
115 calories per serving

Warm Berries & Cream

Ingredients

250g (9oz) blueberries

250g (9oz) strawberries

100g (3½ oz) redcurrants

100g (3½ oz) blackberries

4 tablespoons fresh whipped cream

1 tablespoon honey

Zest and juice of 1 orange

Method

Place all of the berries into a pan along with the honey and orange juice. Gently heat the berries for around 5 minutes until warmed through. Serve the berries into bowls and add a dollop of whipped cream on top. Alternatively you could top them off with fromage frais or yogurt.

Serves 4
180 calories per serving

Chocolate Fondue

Ingredients

125g (4oz) dark chocolate (min 85% cocoa)

300g (11oz) strawberries

200g (7oz) cherries

2 apples, peeled, cored and sliced

100mls (3½ fl oz) double cream (heavy cream)

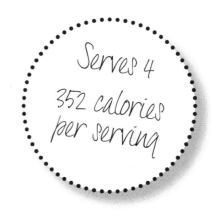

Serves 4
352 calories
per serving

Method

Place the chocolate and cream into a fondue pot or saucepan and warm it until smooth and creamy. Serve in the fondue pot or transfer it to a serving bowl. Scatter the fruit on a serving dish ready to be dipped into the chocolate.

Walnut & Date Loaf

Ingredients

250g (9oz) self-raising flour

125g (4oz) medjool dates, chopped

50g (2oz) walnuts, chopped

250mls (8fl oz) milk

3 eggs

1 medium banana, mashed

1 teaspoon baking soda

Serves 12
166 calories
per serving

Method

Sieve the baking soda and flour into a bowl. Add in the banana, eggs, milk and dates and combine all the ingredients thoroughly. Transfer the mixture to a lined loaf tin and smooth it out. Scatter the walnuts on top. Bake the loaf in the oven at 180C/360F for 45 minutes. Transfer it to a wire rack to cool before serving.

Strawberry Frozen Yogurt

Ingredients

450g (1lb) plain yogurt

175g (6oz) strawberries

Juice of 1 orange

1 tablespoon honey

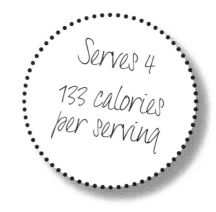

Serves 4
133 calories
per serving

Method

Place the strawberries and orange juice into a food processor or blender and blitz until smooth. Press the mixture through a sieve into a large bowl to remove seeds. Stir in the honey and yogurt. Transfer the mixture to an ice-cream maker and follow the manufacturer's instructions. Alternatively pour the mixture into a container and place in the fridge for 1 hour. Use a fork to whisk it and break up ice crystals and freeze for 2 hours.

Chocolate Brownies

Ingredients

200g (7oz) dark chocolate (min 85% cocoa)

200g (70z) medjool dates, stone removed

100g (3½oz) walnuts, chopped

3 eggs

25mls (1fl oz) melted coconut oil

2 teaspoons vanilla essence

½ teaspoon baking soda

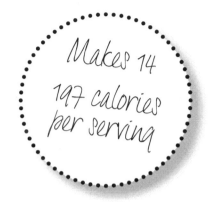

Makes 14
197 calories
per serving

Method

Place the dates, chocolate, eggs, coconut oil, baking soda and vanilla essence into a food processor and mix until smooth. Stir the walnuts into the mixture. Pour the mixture into a shallow baking tray. Transfer to the oven and bake at 180C/350F for 25-30 minutes. Allow it to cool. Cut into pieces and serve.

Crème Brûlée

Ingredients

400g (14oz) strawberries

300g (11oz) plain low fat yogurt

125g (4oz) Greek yogurt

100g (3½oz) brown sugar

1 teaspoon vanilla extract

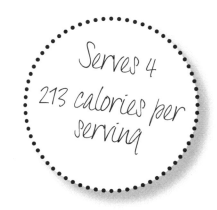

Serves 4
213 calories per serving

Method

Divide the strawberries between 4 ramekin dishes. In a bowl combine the plain yogurt with the vanilla extract. Spoon the mixture onto the strawberries. Scoop the Greek yogurt on top. Sprinkle the sugar into each ramekin dish, completely covering the top. Place the dishes under a hot grill (broiler) for around 3 minutes or until the sugar has caramelised.

Pistachio Fudge

Ingredients

225g (8oz) medjool dates

100g (3½ oz) pistachio nuts, shelled (or other nuts)

50g (2oz) desiccated (shredded) coconut

25g (1oz) oats

2 tablespoons water

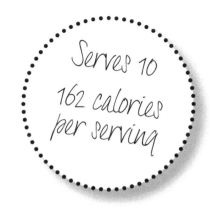

Serves 10
162 calories
per serving

Method

Place the dates, nuts, coconut, oats and water into a food processor and process until the ingredients are well mixed. Remove the mixture and roll it to 2cm (1 inch) thick. Cut it into 10 pieces and serve.

Spiced Poached Apples

Ingredients

4 apples

2 tablespoons honey

4 star anise

2 cinnamon sticks

300mls (½ pint) green tea

Serves 4
99 calories per serving

Method

Place the honey and green tea into a saucepan and bring to the boil. Add the apples, star anise and cinnamon. Reduce the heat and simmer gently for 15 minutes. Serve the apples with a dollop of crème fraiche or Greek yogurt.

Black Forest Smoothie

Ingredients

100g (3½oz) frozen cherries

25g (1oz) kale

1 medjool date

1 tablespoon cocoa powder

2 teaspoons chia seeds

200mls (7fl oz) milk or soya milk

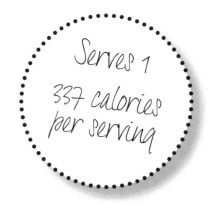

Serves 1
337 calories per serving

Method

Place all the ingredients into a blender and process until smooth and creamy.

Creamy Coffee Smoothie

Ingredients

1 banana

1 teaspoon chia seeds

1 teaspoon coffee

½ avocado

120mls (4fl oz) water

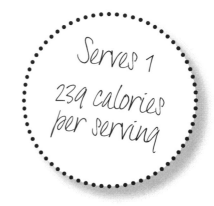

Serves 1
239 calories
per serving

Method

Place all the ingredients into a food processor or blender and blitz until smooth. You can add a little crushed ice too. This can also double as a breakfast smoothie.

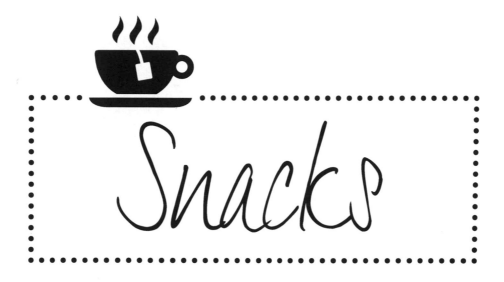

Snacks

Homemade Hummus & Celery

Ingredients

8 sticks of celery, cut into batons

175g (6oz) tinned chickpeas (garbanzo beans), drained

2 cloves of garlic, crushed

1 tablespoon fresh parsley, chopped

1 tablespoon tahini (sesame seed paste)

Juice of 1 lemon

1 tablespoon olive oil

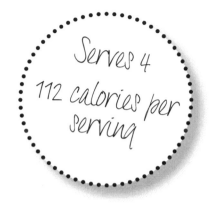

Serves 4
112 calories per serving

Method

Place the chickpeas (garbanzo beans) into a blender along with the garlic, tahini paste and lemon juice. Process until it's smooth and creamy. Transfer the mixture to a serving bowl. Make a small well in the centre of the dip and pour in the olive oil. Sprinkle with parsley. Serve the celery sticks on a plate alongside the hummus.

Pizza Kale Chips

Ingredients

250g (9oz) kale, chopped into approx 4cm (2inch)

50g (2oz) ground almonds

50g (2oz) Parmesan cheese

3 tablespoons tomato purée (tomato paste)

½ teaspoon mixed herbs

½ teaspoon oregano

½ teaspoon onion powder

2 tablespoons olive oil

100mls (3½ fl oz) water

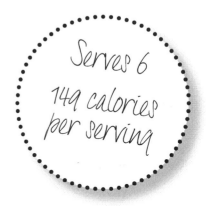

Serves 6
149 calories
per serving

Method

Place all of the ingredients, except the KALE, into food processor and process until finely chopped into a smooth consistency. Toss the kale leaves in the Parmesan mixture, coating it really well. Spread the kale out onto 2 baking sheets. Bake in the oven at 170C/325F for 15 minutes, until crispy.

Rosemary & Garlic Kale Chips

Ingredients

250g (9oz) kale chips, chopped into approx 4cm (2inch)

2 sprigs of rosemary

2 clove of garlic

2 tablespoons olive oil

Sea salt

Freshly ground black pepper

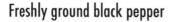

Serves 6
55 calories per serving

Method

Gently warm the olive oil, rosemary and garlic over a low heat for 10 minutes. Remove it from the heat and set aside to cool. Take the rosemary and garlic out of the oil and discard them. Toss the kale leaves in the oil making sure they are well coated. Season with salt and pepper. Spread the kale leaves onto 2 baking sheets and bake them in the oven at 170C/325F for 15 minutes, until crispy.

Honey Chilli Nuts

Ingredients

150g (5oz) walnuts

150g (5oz) pecan nuts

50g (2oz) softened butter

1 tablespoon honey

½ bird's-eye chilli, very finely chopped and de-seeded

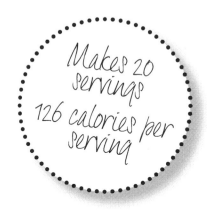

Makes 20 servings
126 calories per serving

Method

Preheat the oven to 180C/360F. Combine the butter, honey and chilli in a bowl then add the nuts and stir them well. Spread the nuts onto a lined baking sheet and roast them in the oven for 10 minutes, stirring once halfway through. Remove from the oven and allow them to cool before eating.

Pomegranate Guacamole

Ingredients

Flesh of 2 ripe avocados

Seeds from 1 pomegranate

1 bird's-eye chilli pepper, finely chopped

½ red onion, finely chopped

Juice of 1 lime

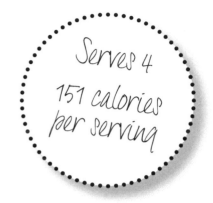

Serves 4
151 calories per serving

Method

Place the avocado, onion, chill and lime juice into a blender and process until smooth. Stir in the pomegranate seeds. Chill before serving. Serve as a dip for chop vegetables.

Tofu Guacamole

Ingredients

225g (8oz) silken tofu

3 avocados

2 tablespoon fresh coriander (cilantro), chopped

1 bird's-eye chilli

Juice of 1 lime

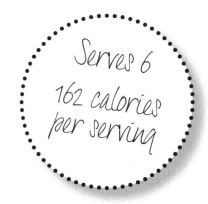

Serves 6
162 calories
per serving

Method

Place all of the ingredients into a food processor and blend a soft chunky consistency. Serve with crudités.

Ginger & Turmeric Tea

Ingredients

2.5cm (1 inch) chunk fresh ginger root, peeled

¼ teaspoon turmeric

1 teaspoon of honey (optional)

Hot water

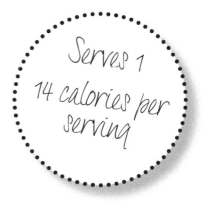

Serves 1
33 calories per serving

Method

Make incisions in the piece of root ginger, without cutting all the way through. Place the ginger and turmeric in a cup and pour in hot water. Allow it to steep for 7 minutes. Add a teaspoon of honey if you wish. Enjoy.

Iced Cranberry Green Tea

Ingredients

150mls (5fl oz) light cranberry juice

100mls (3½ fl oz) green tea, cooled

Squeeze of lemon juice

A handful of crushed ice (optional)

Sprig of mint

Serves 1
14 calories per serving

Method

Pour the green tea and cranberry into a glass and add a squeeze of lemon juice. Top it off with some ice and garnish with a mint leaf.

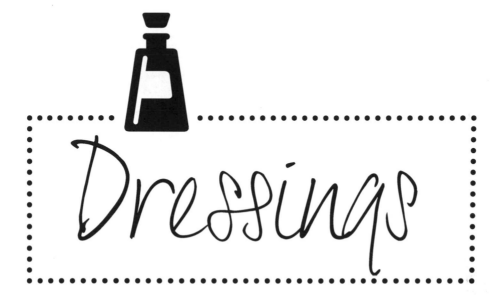

Dressings

Basil & Walnut Pesto

Ingredients

50g (2oz) fresh basil

50g (2oz) walnuts

25g (1oz) pine nuts

3 cloves of garlic, crushed

2 tablespoons Parmesan, grated

4 tablespoons olive oil

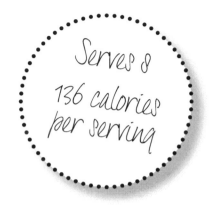

Serves 8
136 calories
per serving

Method

Place the pesto ingredients into a food processor and process until it becomes a smooth paste. Serve with meat, fish, salad and pasta dishes.

Teriyaki Sauce

Ingredients

200mls (7fl oz) soy sauce

200mls (7fl oz) pineapple juice

1 teaspoon red wine vinegar

2.5cm (1 inch) chunk of fresh ginger root, peeled and chopped

2 cloves of garlic

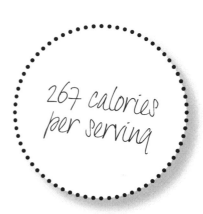

267 calories per serving

Method

Place the ingredients into a saucepan, bring them to the boil, reduce the heat and simmer for 10 minutes. Let it cool then remove the garlic and ginger. Store it in a container in the fridge until ready to use. Use as a marinade for meat, fish and tofu dishes.

Turmeric & Lemon Dressing

Ingredients

1 teaspoon turmeric

4 tablespoons olive oil

Juice of 1 lemon

Method

Combine all the ingredients in bowl and serve with salads. Eat straight away.

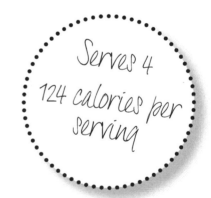

Serves 4
125 calories
per serving

Garlic Vinaigrette

Ingredients

1 clove garlic, crushed

4 tablespoons olive oil

1 tablespoon lemon juice

Freshly ground black pepper

Method

Simply mix all of the ingredients together. It can either be stored or used straight away.

Serves 4
124 calories per
serving

Walnut Vinaigrette

Ingredients

1 clove garlic, finely chopped

6 tablespoons olive oil

3 tablespoons red wine vinegar

1 tablespoon walnut oil

Sea salt

Freshly ground black pepper

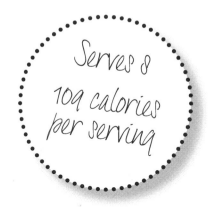

Serves 8
109 calories per serving

Method

Combine all of the ingredients in a bowl or container and season with salt and pepper. Use immediately or store in the fridge.

Walnut & Mint Pesto

Ingredients

6 tablespoons fresh mint leaves

50g (2oz) walnuts

2 cloves of garlic

100g (3½oz) Parmesan cheese

1 tablespoon lemon juice

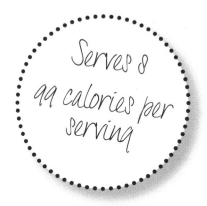

Serves 8
99 calories per serving

Method

Put all the ingredients into a food processor and blend until it becomes a smooth paste.

Parsley Pesto

Ingredients

75g (3½oz) Parmesan cheese, finely grated

50g (2oz) pine nuts

6 tablespoons fresh parsley leaves, chopped

2 cloves of garlic

2 tablespoons olive oil

Serves 8
115 calories per serving

Method

Put all of the ingredients into a food processor or blend until you have a smooth paste.

Lemon Caper Pesto

Ingredients

6 tablespoons fresh parsley leaves

3 cloves of garlic

2 tablespoons capers

50g (2oz) cashew nuts

2 tablespoons olive oil

1 tablespoon lemon juice

Serves 8
95 calories per serving

Method

Place all of the ingredients into a food processor and blitz until smooth. Add a little extra oil if necessary. Serve with pasta, vegetables or meat dishes.

Made in the USA
Monee, IL
31 July 2020